REMEDIES FOR DISEASES

CHANDRIKAA SHARMAA

CHANDRIKAA SHARMAA

Copyright © Chandrikaa Sharmaa
All Rights Reserved.

ISBN 978-1-68509-303-7

This book has been published with all efforts taken to make the material error-free after the consent of the author. However, the author and the publisher do not assume and hereby disclaim any liability to any party for any loss, damage, or disruption caused by errors or omissions, whether such errors or omissions result from negligence, accident, or any other cause.

While every effort has been made to avoid any mistake or omission, this publication is being sold on the condition and understanding that neither the author nor the publishers or printers would be liable in any manner to any person by reason of any mistake or omission in this publication or for any action taken or omitted to be taken or advice rendered or accepted on the basis of this work. For any defect in printing or binding the publishers will be liable only to replace the defective copy by another copy of this work then available.

Contents

1. Acne — 1
2. Allergies — 2
3. Anxiety — 3
4. Arthritis — 4
5. Asthma — 5
6. Back Pain — 6
7. Bad Breath — 7
8. Bed Wetting — 8
9. Body Odour — 9
10. Chapped Lips — 11
11. Coughs — 13
12. Depression — 14
13. Diarrhea — 15
14. Dry Skin — 16
15. Eye Strain — 17
16. Fever — 18
17. Headaches — 20
18. High Blood Pressure — 21
19. High Cholesterol — 22
20. Indigestion — 23
21. Insomnia — 24
22. Kidney Stones — 25
23. Memory Problems — 27
24. Menopause — 29
25. Menstrual Problems — 30
26. Morning Sickness — 32
27. Muscle Cramps — 33
28. Nausea — 35

Contents

29. Neck And Shoulder Pain — 36

30. Oily Skin — 38

31. Pregnancy Ailments — 40

32. Restless Legs Syndrome — 41

33. Sinusitis — 43

34. Snoring — 45

35. Sore Throat — 47

36. Stress — 49

37. Sunburn — 51

38. Toothache — 52

39. Urinary Tract Infections — 54

40. Varicose Veins — 56

41. Water Retention — 57

42. Wind And Flatulence — 59

43. Wrinkles — 61

CHAPTER ONE

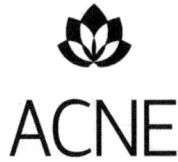

ACNE

Eradicate spots now

- The first avenue of assault is an over-the-counter lotion, liquid or gel formulated with benzoyl peroxide the Oxy range or PanOxyl, for example. These work by mild irritating the skin, which encourages dying skin cells to flake off. This in turn helps to reopen blocked pores. Benzoyl peroxide also kills the bacteria that infect blocked pores.
- Alpha-hydroxy acids (AHAs), such as glycolic acid, slough off the outermost layer of dead skin cells, which helps to keep pores clear and unblocked. Look for any skin cream, lotion or gel that contains glycolic acid.
- At the first hint of a pimple, get out an ice cube, wrap it in a piece of cling film and hold it to the area affected at least twice a day - every hour if you can, but for no longer than five minutes each time. The cold will reduce the redness and ease the inflammation.
- Take aspirin or ibuprofen. These painkillers are anti- inflammatory and can help to calm an acne outbreak. Take the recommended adult dose up to four times a day. (Do not take aspirin regularly for more than a few days without checking with your doctor, and never give aspirin to a child under 16.)

CHAPTER TWO

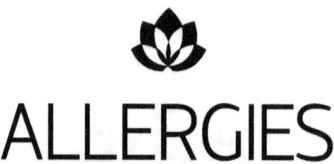

ALLERGIES

Nature's antihistamines

- Nettle contains a substance that works as a antihistamine. Capsules of the freeze-dried leaf are health-food shops. Take 500mg three times a day.
- Ginkgo biloba has become renowned for its memory boosting properties, but it can also be an effective allery fighter. Ginkgo contains substances called ginkgolides, which can halt the activity of certain allergy-triggering chemicals (platelet activating factor, or PAF). Take up to 240mg a day.
- Quercetin, the pigment that gives grapes their purple hue and puts the green in green tea, inhibits the release of histamine. Take one 500mg capsule twice a day. (Alert Do not take this if already taking nettle, as nettle contains quercetin.)
- **Try something fishy**
- Omega-3 fatty acids help to counter inflammatory responses in the body, such as those triggered by allergies. Salmon, sardines, fresh tuna and mackerel are good sources of these fats. If you prefer the idea of fish oil capsules, take a supplement that provides 1000mg combined EPA/DHA (eicosapentaenoic and docosahexanoic acids) a day.
- Flax seed oil (or linseed oil) is another excellent source of omega-3 fatty acids. Take 1 tablespoon of flax seed oil a day. You can add it to salad dressing or a glass of juice or blend it into a smoothie, but avoid heating it.

CHAPTER THREE

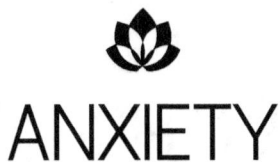

ANXIETY

Soak away your cares

- A warm bath is one of the most pleasant and reliable ways to soothe your senses. To enhance its effects, add some lavender oil (or dried flowers if you have them) to the tub and soak to your heart's content. Although no one knows what gives this wonderfully scented herb its ability to calm, lavender has been used for around 2,000 years to relax and soothe the nerves. If you have no time for a bath, try dabbing a little lavender oil on your temples and forehead and sitting quietly for a few minutes. Breathe slowly and deeply
- Regulating your breath can help to bring your anxiety swiftly under control. To slow and deepen your breathing, sit down, put one hand over your abdomen, and slowly inhale so that your belly expands under your hand but your shoulders do not rise. Hold your breath for four or five seconds, then very slowly exhale. Repeat until you feel calmer.

CHAPTER FOUR

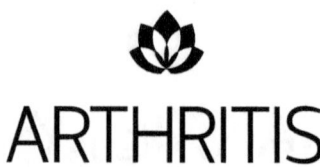

ARTHRITIS

Pain removers

- Take glucosamine and chondroitin sulphate supplements to reduce pain and slow down cartilage loss. Evidence suggests that this combination can be effective for people with mild to moderate arthritis. Follow the dosage directions on the label, and persevere: it may take a month or more before you begin to feel the benefits.
- Take a teaspoon of powdered ginger or up to 35g (about 6 teaspoons) of fresh ginger once a day. Research shows that ginger root helps to relieve arthritis pain, probably because of its ability to increase blood circulation, and thus ferry inflammatory chemicals away from painful joints.
- Take two 400mg doses of SAM-e (S-adenosylmethionine) a day. Supplementing with SAM-e, a chemical found naturally in all cells of the body, has been shown to help relieve arthritis pain by increasing blood levels of proteoglycans – molecules that seem to play a key role in preserving cartilage by helping to keep it 'plumped up' and well oxygenated. SAM-e also appears to reduce inflammation. Research has found the supplement as effective as anti-inflammatory drugs such as ibuprofen in fighting arthritis pain.
- If you get good results with 800mg a day, reduce the dose to 400mg a day after two weeks. SAM-e has few side-effects, although it can cause dyspepsia and nausea. It seems to be safe to take with most prescription and OTC drugs, but if you are taking drugs prescribed for bipolar disorder (manic depression) or Parkinson's disease, you should consult your doctor before taking SAM-e supplements.

CHAPTER FIVE

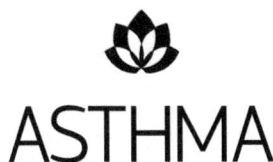

ASTHMA

Ease breathing during an attack

- When an asthma attack occurs, try to stay calm. Panic can make your symptoms worse. This visualization trick may help. Close your eyes. As you inhale, see your lungs expand and fill with white light and feel your breathing become easier. Repeat this exercise twice more, then open your eyes.
- In an emergency, drink a strong cup of coffee, two 330ml cans of cola or a Red Bull or Lipovitan (both of which are high in caffeine). Caffeine is chemically related to theophylline, a medication for asthma. It helps to open the airways.

Combat constriction with supplements

- Practitioners of traditional Chinese medicine have been using the herb ginkgo to treat asthma for centuries. One recent study suggests that this herb interferes with a protein in the blood that contributes to airway spasms. If you want to try it, buy supplements labelled ginkgo biloba extract, or GBE, and take up to 250mg a day.
- Magnesium may make you feel better. Much research suggests that magnesium relaxes the airways. The recommended dose is 300mg a day for men and 270mg for women.

CHAPTER SIX

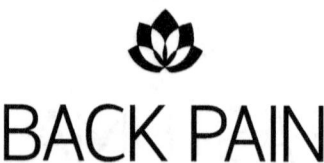

BACK PAIN

Ice first, heat later

- As a pain reliever, ice works really well. It temporarily blocks pain signals and helps to reduce swelling. Several times a day, place an ice pack wrapped in a towel on the painful area for up to 20 minutes. Alternatively, you can use a bag of frozen peas. During the first few days of home treatment, apply the ice pack as often as necessary. Later, you may still want to use ice after exercise or any physical activity.
- After about 48 hours, switch to moist heat to stimulate blood flow and reduce painful spasms. Dip a towel in very warm water, wring it out, then flatten and fold it. Lie on your stomach with pillows under your hips and ankles. Place the towel across the painful area, cover the towel with cling film, then put a heating pad - set on medium - on top of the film. Leave it on for up to 20 minutes. You can repeat this three or four times a day for several days.

Rub in some relief

- Ask a partner or close friend to massage the aching area. If you want to use a cream or ointment sold as a 'back rub', then do so, but with care - these topical creams tend to cause skin irritation after a few applications. For a simple back-massage aid, stuff several tennis balls into a long sock, tie the end of the sock, and ask your partner to roll it up and down your back.

CHAPTER SEVEN

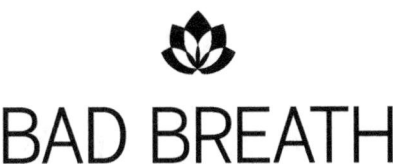

BAD BREATH

Take emergency measures

- A dry mouth is a haven for the bacteria that cause bad breath. So find a tap and swish the water around in your th Water will temporarily dislodge bacteria and make your breath a bit more acceptable.
- At the end of your business lunch or romantic dinner. munch the sprig of parsley that's left on your plate. Parsley is rich in chlorophyll, a well known breath deodorizer with germ- fighting properties.
- If you can get hold of an orange, peel and eat it. The citric acid it contains will stimulate your salivary glands and encourage the flow of breath-freshening saliva.
- If there are no oranges in sight, eat whatever is available, except known breath-pollutants such as garlic, onions or a stinky cheese. Eating encourages the flow of saliva, which helps to remove the unpleasant, odour-causing material on the surface of your tongue.
- Vigorously scrape your tongue over your teeth. Your tongue can become coated with bacteria that ferment proteins, producing gases that smell bad. Scraping your tongue can dislodge these bacteria so you can rinse them away.
- If you have a metal or plastic spoon to hand, you can use it as an effective tongue scraper. To scrape safely, place the spoon on the back of your tongue and drag it forwards. Repeat four live times. Scrape the sides of the tongue as well, with the same back-to-front motion. But don't push the spoon too far back in your mouth as you may activate your gag, reflex and cause yourself to vomit.

CHAPTER EIGHT

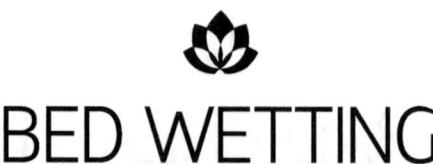

BED WETTING

Keep those 'wee hours' drier

- Restrict your child's fluid intake for an hour before h In particular, cut out cola drinks or hot chocolate that may contain caffeine, which irritates the bladder.
- If your child usually drinks a mug of milk at bedtime, try to stop the practice for a week or two and see if it helps. A few children are allergic to the proteins in milk, primarily casein and whey, and the allergy can cause bedwetting.
- Make sure your child goes to the toilet before he or she goes to bed. It won't stop the bedwetting, but there will be less stored urine, which means less urine to wet the bed.
- Make the pre-bedtime routine calm and quiet. Rough, active play or even an exciting television programme increases the risk of bedwetting. Read a story or leave the child to read alone in bed.
- If the child is seven or older, consider buying a bedwetting alarm. This is a battery operated sensor that emits a buzzing ringing sound when it detects moisture. It conditions children to recognize the need to urinate and wake up before they have to go. Don't give up if the alarm hasn't solved the problem a after week or two; most children respond within two months.

CHAPTER NINE

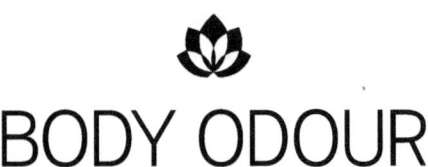

BODY ODOUR

Choose an effective soap

- Pick a deodorant soap, such as Wright's Coal Tar, tea tree soap (from Holland & Barrett) or anti-bacterial hand-washes, such as Boots, Carex or supermarket own brands. These leave ingredients on your skin that continue to kill bacteria even after you've finished washing. If the soap doesn't irritate your skin, use it every day. Some people find these soaps too drying, in which case their use should be restricted to the underarms and groin, where they are needed most.
- If deodorant soap doesn't do the trick, then bring out the big guns. Antibacterial surgical scrubs, such as Hibiscrub or Betadine, are available over-the-counter in most pharmacies. These are so effective that they are used to clean patients before surgery. But as these products can dry your skin, you should use them only in the shower, so you can rinse off quickly, and only on high-smell areas such as the armpits and groin. Squeeze out a little of the cleanser, wash the target areas, then rinse off and finish your shower with ordinary soap.

Beyond deodorant

- Use a cotton wool pad to wipe vinegar onto your armpits during the day to cut down the numbers of odour-causing bacteria. Don't use immediately after shaving, though, or it will sting badly. The same applies to witch hazel (below).
- Dab on witch hazel. You can splash it directly onto your skin or apply it as often as you like with a cotton wool pad. The refreshing, clean-smelling liquid is both drying and deodorizing.

- Dust bicarbonate of soda or cornflour on any problem part of your body. Both of these powders absorb moisture, and bicarb also kills odour-causing bacteria.

CHAPTER TEN

CHAPPED LIPS

Bring out the lip balm

- One all-natural salve is beeswax, such as Burs Beeswax lip balm, sold in pharmacies. Always coat your lips with balm before you go out to keep the elements at bay.
- Some people swear by cocoa butter to relieve chapped lips (It also works on chapped hands.) Apply four or five times a day, or more often if your lips are very dry.
- A handy home remedy is olive oil or vegetable shortening which can effectively soften and moisturize chapped lips.
- If you have vitamin E capsules to hand, puncture one and apply the oil to your lips.
- Petroleum jelly, such as Vaseline, is an old-fashioned and effective chapped lips remedy.
- The label on one US brand of udder cream says that it's for cows but that most of its users have two legs. That's because it's so effective for chapped lips. Various products are available here but look for any formulated with lanolin and petrolatum (the stuff in petroleum jelly). You may find them in some country stores or you can order them online,

Moisturize from the inside out

If your lips are continually chapped, drink eight 250ml glasses of water a day - more, if you can. While this won't prevent dryness, it will keep it from getting worse.

The power of prevention

Apply a balm with a sun protection factor (SPF) of a least 15 before you go out into the sun. Lips need just as much sun protection as the rest of your skin. (Alert Stop using the balm if your lips turn red and itchy. Some people have an allergic reaction to lip balms that contain sunscreen.)

CHAPTER ELEVEN

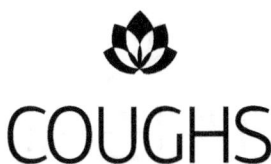

COUGHS

Suck something soothing

- Suck any cough drops or boiled sweets. The hard sweet increases saliva production and causes you to swallow more suppressing coughs.
- For 'productive' coughs, try white horehound. A bittersweet herb, it acts as an expectorant, triggering the coughing reflex and helping to bring up phlegm. Potters produce a horehound and aniseed cough mixture, available in pharmacies.
- For 'dry coughs, try and get hold of slippery elm lozenges (sold online and in some health-food shops). Made from the bark of the slippery elm tree, these were once medicine-chest staples. Slippery elm is loaded with a gel-like substance that coats the throat and keeps coughing to a minimum.

Dose a cough with homemade syrups

- Blend 2 tablespoons lemon juice with 1 tablespoon honey and add a pinch of cayenne pepper. The honey coats your throat, soothing irritated tissues, while the lemon reduces inflammation and delivers a dose of infection-fighting vitamin C. The cayenne boosts circulation in the area, hastening the healing process. Or, instead of cayenne, add a little freshly grated onion. Onions contain irritating compounds that trigger the cough reflex and bring up phlegm.
- Another onion remedy is to peel and chop 6 medium onions and put them with 4 tablespoons of honey into a bowl set over a pan of boiling water (or a double boiler). Cover and simmer for 2 hours. Strain the mixture and take 1 tablespoon every 2 or 3 hours.

CHAPTER TWELVE

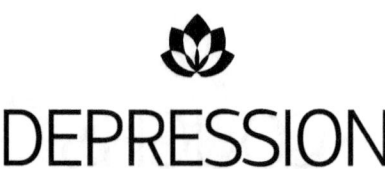

DEPRESSION

Look to food to change your mood

- If you're on a high-protein diet to lose weight, lack of carbohydrates could be contributing to your miserable mood. Foods like fruits, vegetables, beans and whole grains help your brain to make the mood-regulating brain chemical serotonin.
- Aim to eat fish three times a week or more. Researchers in Finland found that people who ate fish less than once a week had a 31 per cent higher incidence of mild to moderate depression than people who ate fish more often. Fresh tuna, salmon, sardines and mackerel are top choices; they're rich in omega-3 fatty acids, essential to normal brain function. There's early evidence that they also influence serotonin production.
- If you drink coffee or cola, cut back or even give it up. Caffeine suppresses serotonin production and has been linked to depression.
- Avoid alcohol. While wine, beer or spirits may initially lift your mood, alcohol is actually a depressant.

CHAPTER THIRTEEN

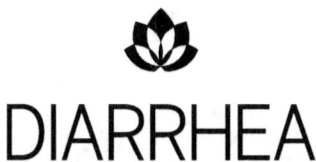

DIARRHEA

Tame diarrhea with tannins

- Drink black tea with sugar. Tea will rehydrate the body contains astringent tannins that help to reduce intestinal inflammation and block the absorption of toxins by intestines. The sugar improves sodium and water absorption
- Tannin-rich blackberries have long been used in full remedies for diarrhoea. To make blackberry tea place 1.5 of dried blackberry leaves in a cup of boiling water; leave to infuse for 10 minutes and strain. Take 3 cups a day between meals. Or bring 2 tablespoons of fresh blackberries to the boil in 250ml water, simmer gently for 10 minutes, then strain. Drink 1 cup several times a day. You can also buy blackberry tea bags in health-food shops; check that they contain blackberry leaves. Raspberry leaf tea is also said to be effective. It is rich in minerals and some vitamins. It's widely used in pregnancy but possibly best avoided in the early stages (up to about 12 weeks).

Root out the problem

- Capsules of goldenseal, made from the bright-yellow room of a perennial herb, appear to kill many of the bacteria, such E. coli, that cause diarrhoea. The key compound in the herb is berberine, which is so effective that goldenseal is sometimes called a 'herbal antibiotic'. Take two or three 125mg caps day until the diarrhoea subsides.

CHAPTER FOURTEEN

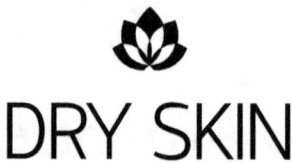

DRY SKIN

Exfoliate for softer skin

- Give your skin a milk bath. The lactic acid in milk exfoliates dead skin cells and may also increase the skin's ability to hold in moisture. Soak a flannel in cold milk. Lay the flannel on any area of skin that is particularly dry or irritated. Leave it there for 5 minutes and when you rinse off the milk, do so gently, so some of the lactic acid stays on your skin.
- To soften rough patches of skin, fill a bath with warm water and add 2 cups of Epsom salts, then climb in and soak for a few minutes. While your skin is still wet, you can also rub handfuls of Epsom salts on the rough areas to exfoliate the skin. You'll be amazed at just how good your skin feels when you get out. If you have any dried seaweed, you can also add a few strips to your bath to boost the softening effect.
- Apply aloe vera gel to help your dry skin heal more quickly. It contains acids that eat away dead skin cells. To obtain the fresh gel, cut off a leaf at the base and split it open with a knife. Scrape out the gel with a spoon.
- Use a moisturizer that contains alpha-hydroxy acids (AHAs) or a lotion that contains urea, such as Eucerin. These remove loose, flaky skin cells, leaving the skin softer.

CHAPTER FIFTEEN

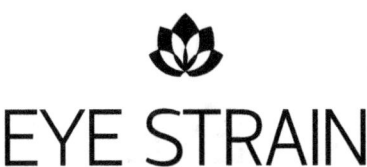

EYE STRAIN

Rest them, blink them, close them

- Whenever you're working on a task that requires close concentration, take a break every 20 minutes or so. Look at a faraway object - a picture on the opposite wall or a view out of the window - for at least 30 seconds. By allowing your eyes to shift focus, you give them a rest.
- Try to blink often - every few seconds or so - when you're paying close attention to your television or computer screen. Blinking moistens your eyeballs and relaxes your eye muscles.
- If you have a long task that involves prolonged staring, close your eyes periodically. Even if you just shut your eyelids for a few seconds, you'll get some immediate relief.

Warm and cool relief

- Another way to relax your eye muscles: Briskly rub your hands together until they grow warm, and gently place the heels of your palms over your closed eyes. Hold them there for a few seconds.
- If you soak a flannel or hand towel in cool water, wring it out, and lay it over your eyes for 5 minutes to relieve strain.
- Cool your eyes with sliced cucumber. Lie on your back and place a slice over each closed eye. Leave on for 2 or 3 minutes, or replace the first pair with another, cooler set of slices.

CHAPTER SIXTEEN

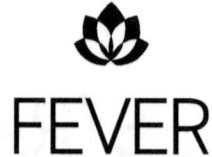

FEVER

Be cool

- Take a bath in lukewarm water. This temperature will feel pretty cool when you have a fever and the bath should help to bring your body temperature down. Don't try to bring a fever down rapidly by plunging yourself into cold water; that will send blood rushing to your internal organs, which is how the body defends itself from cold. Your interior actually warms up instead of cooling down.
- Give yourself a sponge bath. Tepid sponging of high-heat areas like the armpits and groin with cool water can help to reduce a temperature as the water evaporates.
- When you're not bathing, place cold, damp flannels on your forehead and the back of your neck.

Sweat it out

- Brew a cup of yarrow tea. This herb opens your pores and triggers sweating, helping to move a fever on. Steep a tablespoon of the herb in a cup of boiling water for 10 minutes. Let it cool and strain. Drink a cup or two until you start to sweat.
- Another herb, elderflower, also helps you to sweat. And it happens to be good for other problems associated with flu and colds, like overproduction of mucus. To make elderflower tea, mix 2 teaspoons of the herb in a cup of boiling water and let it steep for 15 minutes. Strain out the elderflower. Drink three times a day as long as the fever continues.
- Drink a cup of hot ginger tea, which also induces sweating. To make the tea, steep ½ teaspoon of minced root ginger in a cup of boiling water.

Strain, then drink.

CHAPTER SEVENTEEN

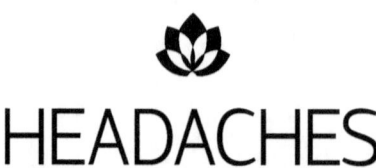

HEADACHES

Give it some acupressure

- With a firm, circular motion, massage the web of skin between the base of your thumb and your forefinger. Continue massaging for several minutes, then switch hands and repeat until the pain clears up. Acupressure experts call this fleshy area trigger point LIG4 and maintain that it is linked to areas of the brain where headaches originate.

Heat up and cool down

- Believe it or not, soaking your feet in hot water will help your head to feel better. By drawing blood to your feet, the hot-water footbath will ease pressure on the blood vessels in your head. For a really bad headache, add a bit of mustard powder to the water.
- For a tension headache, place a hot compress on your forehead or the back on your neck. The heat will help to relax knotted-up muscles in this area.
- It might sound contradictory, but you can follow up the heat treatment (or substitute it) by applying a cold compress to your forehead. Wrap a couple of ice cubes in a flannel or use a bag of frozen peas wrapped in a tea towel. Cold constricts blood vessels and, when they shrink, they stop pressing on sensitive nerves. Because headache pain sometimes originates in the nerves in the back of your neck, try moving the compress to the muscles at the base of your skull.
- Here's an alternative to a cold compress: soak your hands in iced water for as long as you can stand it. While your hands are submerged in the water, repeatedly open and close your

CHAPTER EIGHTEEN

HIGH BLOOD PRESSURE

Start tackling the problem in the kitchen

- Studies in the USA have shown that a diet known as DASH (short for Dietary Approaches to Stop Hypertension) is very effective at lowering blood pressure. The gist of the diet is this: it's low in saturated fat and cholesterol and high in fruit, vegetables, whole grains and low-fat dairy foods. A diet based on these principals can produce positive results - a reduction in blood pressure - in as little as two weeks.
- Reduce your salt intake. Eating too much salt causes your body to retain water. The effect is the same as adding more liquid to an overfilled water balloon: pressure rises. In a follow up to the DASH study, researchers found that the biggest drop in blood pressure came when people followed the DASH diet and also limited themselves to 1500mg of sodium a day. That's less than a teaspoon of salt a day.
- Even if you don't add salt to your food during cooking or at the table, you may still be getting a considerable amount of 'hidden' salt in packaged and processed foods, especially snacks, meat products and tinned soups. So before buying food, read labels carefully to find out the sodium or salt content. Look for low-salt soups and biscuits and rinse beans and other foods canned in brine before using them. . Try making your own bread. If you have a bread maker, it takes less than 5 minutes a day to tip in the ingredients and, 2 hours later, there's the bread. Why bother? Because most shop bread contains high levels of salt, and you can control exactly how much salt - and fat - goes into a homemade loaf. And it's delicious and makes the house smell wonderful.

CHAPTER NINETEEN

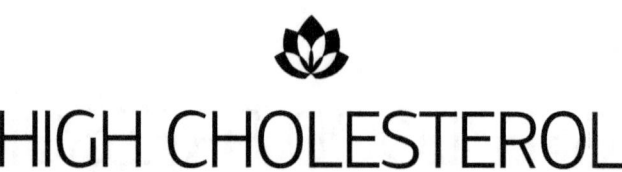

HIGH CHOLESTEROL

Cut out the 'bad' fats

- Eliminate as much saturated fat as possible from your diet. That means switching to leaner cuts of meats and lower-fat versions of dairy products such as butter, milk, ice cream, cheese and yoghurt. Cut out processed meats - such as salami, corned beef and pork pie - altogether.
- Run screaming from palm oil and coconut oil, which are very high in saturated fat. These so-called tropical oils are found in many processed foods, particularly biscuits and cakes.
- Another type of fat, called trans-fatty acids should be avoided as much as possible. They are produced when plant-based oils are hydrogenated to produce solid spreads, such as margarines. They have the same effect on cholesterol levels as saturated fat. Many shop-bought cakes, biscuits, snack foods - and even breads - are loaded with these fats. To find them, look for the word 'hydrogenated on the list of ingredients.
- Eat more fresh fruits, vegetables and whole grains. That is the easiest way to feel full as you cut back on meat and other fatty foods. In addition to being low in fat and cholesterol-free, plant foods contain lots of cholesterol-lowering fibre and vitamins and antioxidants that are good for your heart.
- If you love dark meat, try venison. This game meat has a fraction of the fat found in most of the beef that is sold in supermarkets. In fact, it is as low in fat as most fish. Marinate venison to improve its tenderness.

CHAPTER TWENTY

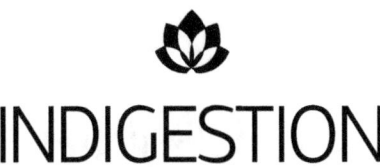

INDIGESTION

Well-rooted in tradition

- Ginger has long been used for settling stomach upsets and quelling nausea. No one is quite sure how it works, but it has been shown to improve digestion and it has antispasmodic properties, which makes it a helpful remedy for stomach cramps. Ginger is easily taken in capsule form: take two 250mg capsules after food. Or follow a meal with a few pieces of candied root ginger or a tummy-warming cup of ginger tea. To make the tea, stir a teaspoon of fresh grated ginger root into a cup of boiling water, steep for 10 minutes and strain.
- Camomile is an age-old treatment for indigestion. The herb is best taken as a soothing tea - widely available in sachets from health food stores and supermarkets. Drink 3 cups of camomile tea a day, before meals.

Pamper yourself with peppermint

- Peppermint oil soothes intestinal cramps and helps to relieve abdominal bloating. It is best taken as slow release capsules such as Colpermin or Mintec. Take 1 or 2 capsules three times a day after food. Or you could try Obbekjaers peppermint oil capsules, available from health food stores or online. Take 1 capsule three times a day, with a little water, before meals. (Alert If you have heartburn, peppermint is not the best cure for you - it can make acid reflux problems worse. Avoid taking indigestion remedies at the same time of day as peppermint oil. If you take cyclosporine (a drug for rheumatoid arthritis), check with your doctor before taking peppermint oil.)

CHAPTER TWENTY-ONE

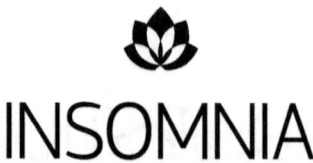

INSOMNIA

Bedtime snacks

- Have a slice of turkey or chicken or a banana before going to bed. These foods contain tryptophan, an amino acid that the body uses to make serotonin. And serotonin is a brain chemical that helps you to sleep. Keep the helping small, though, or your full tummy may keep you awake.
- Carbohydrates help trytophan to enter the brain. Try a glass of warm milk (milk contains tryptophan) and a biscuit, or warm milk with a spoonful of honey. A sprinkling of cinnamon won't hurt and might add mild sedative properties of its own.
- Avoid large meals late in the evening. You need three to four hours to digest a big meal, so if you eat a lot within three hours of your bedtime, don't be surprised if intestinal grumblings and groanings keep you awake.
- Spicy or sugary food, even at suppertime, is usually a bad idea. Spices can irritate your stomach, and when it tosses and turns, so will you. Having a lot of sugary food - especially chocolate, which contains caffeine - can make you feel jumpy.

CHAPTER TWENTY-TWO

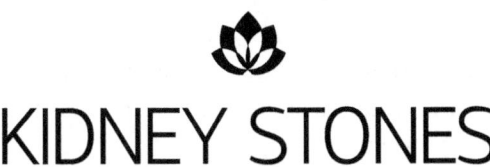

KIDNEY STONES

Flush it out

- To flush the stone into the bladder, drink at least three litres of water a day. If you're gulping enough water to do the job, your urine should run clear, with not a trace of yellow.
- During an attack, drink as much dandelion tea as you can A strong diuretic, dandelion stimulates blood circulation through the kidneys, increasing urine output and helping to flush out the stone. To make the tea, add 2 teaspoons dried herb to 1 cup boiling water. Steep for 15 minutes, then drink.
- Consider drinking 2 or 3 cups a day of buchu tea. Like dandelion, this herb has diuretic properties which may help to flush out and prevent kidney stones. Place a sachet (2g) of buchu into a cup of boiling water and drink 1 cup three times a day before meals.

Stepping stone

- When you have a kidney stone, the slightest move is likely to be painful. But if you can bear to take a walk, try to do so. Walking may jar the stone loose. Despite the discomfort, you might pass the stone more quickly if you just keep moving. The power of prevention
- Many experts believe that the single most important thing you can do to prevent kidney stones is the same thing you do to make them pass more quickly - that is, drink enough fluids. Anyone who is prone to kidney stones should drink at least 8 to 10 cups of water a day, every day. The more you drink, the more you dilute the substances that form stones.
- Stick to a low-salt diet to reduce the calcium in your urine, which may reduce your risk of forming new stones.

- A good start is to limit your consumption of fast foods, tinned soups and other processed foods. Read labels carefully. The target is less than 6g salt (2,400mg sodium) a day
- Drink two 250ml glasses of cranberry juice each day. Research suggests that it may help to reduce the amount of calcium in the urine. In one study of people with calcium stones, cranberry juice reduced the amount of calcium in the urine by 50 per cent.
- If you don't like cranberry juice, drink orange juice or real lemonade - 200ml (⅜ pint) at each meal. The citric acid these juices contain will raise the citrate level in your urine, helping to keep new calcium stones from forming.
- Magnesium has been shown to prevent all types of kidney stones. Eat more foods rich in this mineral, such as dark-green leafy vegetables, wheatgerm and seafood. You can also take 300mg a day in supplement form.
- Boost your intake of fruits and vegetables - especially bananas, oranges and orange juice, which are rich in potassium. In studies, people who ate a lot of fresh produce slashed their risk of kidney stones by half. If you suffer from stones regularly, ask your doctor whether potassium supplements might help you to ward off future attacks.
- Cut back on coffee. Caffeine increases calcium in the urine, which increases the risk of stone formation.
- If you know your stones are made of calcium oxalate (a urine test can tell you), cut back on foods rich in oxalates. These foods include rhubarb, spinach, chocolate, wheat bran, nuts (especially peanuts), strawberries and raspberries. Also avoid drinking tea, which is high in oxalates.

CHAPTER TWENTY-THREE

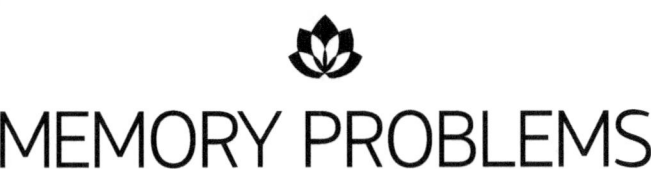

MEMORY PROBLEMS

Catch the scent

- Buy a small bottle of either rosemary or basil essential oil from a health-food shop. Tests of brain waves show that inhaling either of these scents increases the brain's production of beta waves, which indicate heightened awareness. All you need to do is put a trace of the oil in your hair, wrists or clothing - anywhere you can get a whiff. Or put some of the oil in a diffuser and let it fill the air.

Count on coffee

- If you drink caffeinated drinks, you'll get a short-term boost in your ability to concentrate. And there may be long-term benefits as well. At the Faculty of Medicine in Lisbon, Portugal, researchers found that elderly people who drank 3 or 4 cups of coffee a day were less likely to experience memory loss than people who drank a cup a day or less.

Give it oxygen

- Take 120mg of ginkgo biloba a day. The herb appears to improve blood flow to the brain, which helps brain cells to get the oxygen they need to perform at their peak. In Germany, where the government's Commission E reports regularly on the effectiveness of herbal medicines, a standardized extract of ginkgo is frequently prescribed to prevent memory loss as well as stroke. If you're perfectly healthy, you probably won't see any beneficial effect from ginkgo. But if you have diminished blood flow to the brain, it may help.

- Another way to increase the flow of blood to the brain is to get moving. There's even some evidence that exercise may

CHAPTER TWENTY-FOUR

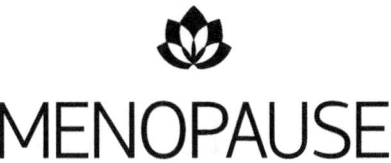

MENOPAUSE

Say 'yes' to soya

- Eat 200mg tofu every day. Tofu is high in phytoestrogens – compounds with mild oestrogen-like qualities that have been found to ease menopausal symptoms. Certain kinds of phytoestrogens, called isoflavones, found in soya products can help to ease hot flushes and vaginal dryness. The recommended amount is 60mg a day of isoflavones, which is what you'll get by eating 200mg of tofu.
- One 50mg supplement of isoflavones, taken daily, can meet most of your needs if you can't face eating tofu every day. Look for brands that contain genistein and daidzein.
- Flax seeds are another source of phytoestrogens. Grind some in a spice mill or coffee grinder and add 1 to 2 tablespoons to cereal or yoghurt.

Ease night sweats

- To help control hot flushes and night sweats, take up to 1ml of black cohosh in tincture form two to four times a day. To make it more palatable, add the tincture to half a glass of juice or water. Research has shown that the herb helps to control hot flushes by lowering blood levels of luteinizing hormone (LH), which dilates blood vessels and sends heat to the skin. You might get other benefits as well, as some women have found that black cohosh relieves vaginal dryness, nervousness and depression. For maximum effectiveness, take black cohosh for six weeks, then take four weeks off before resuming it again. Then repeat the cycle - six weeks on, four weeks off.
- To tame night sweats, take 3 to 15 drops sage tincture three times a day in half a cup of water or tea. The genus name of

CHAPTER TWENTY-FIVE

MENSTRUAL PROBLEMS

Take anti-cramp action

- When you feel cramps coming on, go for a walk or run. Or go swimming. Or get on an exercise bike. Any kind of exercise helps to inhibit prostaglandin production and boosts the release of painkilling endorphins. As a bonus, exercise can also help to relieve bloating.
- Soak in a hot bath. The warmth helps to relax knotted-up muscles in the uterus. Or lie down with a hot-water bottle or heating pad on your abdomen.
- Try a homeopathic remedy. For severe cramps experts recommend mag phos (phosphate of magnesia). Take five pellets of 6C or 12C every hour for five doses. If the cramps don't improve, take the same dosage of pulsatilla or nux vomica. Pulsatilla is advised when you find yourself not only cramping, but crying as well while nux vomica is usually recommended for cramps accompanied by constipation and extreme irritability. Tame cramps with tea
- During the day, drink 3 cups of warm red raspberry-lear tea. (Look for raspberry-leaf tea bags at the supermarket or a health- food shop.) The leaves contain fragrine, a substance that tones the uterus and helps to ease cramping. It can also lighten excessive bleeding.
- As its name implies, cramp bark (Viburnum opulus) can take the edge off cramps. Buy the dried bark (usually available at health-shops) and make a tea using 1 teaspoon bark in 1 cup water, or buy the tincture and follow the dosage directions on the label.
- Good old camomile tea has antispasmodic properties to unclench your uterus. Use 2 to 4 teaspoons of herb per cup of hot water, or buy camomile tea bags. Peppermint is another antispasmodic herb.

- Ginger is another tried and trusted cramp remedy. It is thought to work by inhibiting the production of prostaglandins. To make ginger tea, grate 1 teaspoon fresh root ginger, add a cup boiling water, steep for 10 minutes, then strain.

CHAPTER TWENTY-SIX

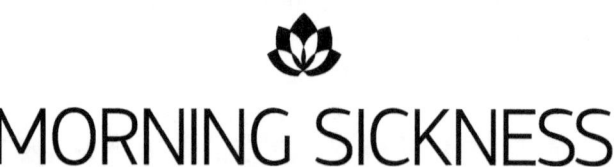

MORNING SICKNESS

Give your tummy a treat

- Nothing beats morning sickness like a cup of ginger tea. The same spicy herb is used to counter motion sickness. To make ginger tea, use a ginger teabag, available in health-food shops and supermarkets, or add teaspoon grated root ginger to 1 cup of very hot water, leave to infuse for 5 minutes, strain and sip.
- Herbal teas made with camomile, lemon balm and peppermint are also known to reduce nausea. Use 1 to 2 teaspoons of the dried herb per cup of hot water. Avoid peppermint tea if you have heartburn, however.
- Brew yourself a cup of raspberry-leaf tea. The herb is used to help with morning sickness - and a lot of women drink it in gradually increasing doses in later pregnancy to ease labour because it acts as a uterine tonic. Use 1 to 2 teaspoons of the dried herb per cup of hot water. Drink no more than 1 cup a day in the first three months of pregnancy (and avoid raspberry leaf tablets). Some people advise that raspberry leaf shouldn't be taken in early pregnancy and should be avoided by women at risk of miscarriage or premature labour but there appears to be no scientific evidence of ill-effects, despite widespread worldwide use for centuries. However, to be on the safe side, consult your midwife or doctor.
- Drink flat, room-temperature ginger ale to settle your stomach. Although no one knows why (there's not enough ginger in shop- bought ginger ale to have an effect), it works for many nauseated mums-to-be. Don't drink ginger ale with

CHAPTER TWENTY-SEVEN

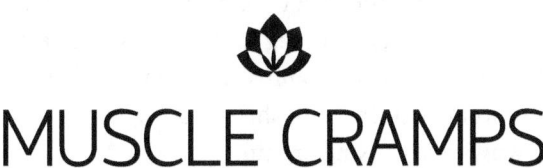

MUSCLE CRAMPS

Put the heat on

- Place an electric heating pad or a hot flannel on the misbehaving muscle to relax the cramp and increase blood flow to the affected tissue. Set the pad on low, apply for 20 minutes then remove it for at least 20 minutes before reapplying.
- Take a long, warm shower or soak in the bath. For added relief, pour in half a cup of Epsom salts. The magnesium in Epsom salts promotes muscle relaxation.

Press out pain

- Find the central point of the cramp. Press this spot with your thumb, the heel of your hand or a loosely clenched fist. Hold the pressure for 10 seconds, ease off for 10 seconds, then press again. You should feel some discomfort but not excruciating pain. After several repetitions, the pain should start to diminish.

Rub it in

- Mix 1 part oil of wintergreen (available from chemists or essential oils suppliers) with 4 parts vegetable oil and massage it into the cramp. Wintergreen contains methyl salicylate (related to aspirin), which relieves pain and stimulates bloodflow. You can use this mixture several times a day, but with a heating pad - you could burn your skin. (Alert NO that wintergreen is highly toxic by mouth.)

Banish night-time leg cramps

- Before bed, drink a glass of tonic water, which con quinine, a popular remedy for leg cramps. Research has supported the use of quinine for nocturnal leg cramps, but don't take quinine tablets, they can have serious side effects, such as ringing in the cars and disturbed vision,
- To prevent night-time calf cramps, try not to sleep with your toes pointed. And don't tuck in your sheets too tightly - this tends to bend your toes downwards, causing cramp.
- Take 250mg vitamin E a day to prevent nocturnal leg cramps. Studies suggest that taking vitamin E improves bloodflow through the arteries.

CHAPTER TWENTY-EIGHT

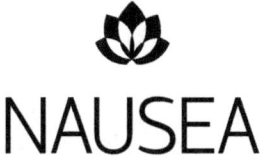

NAUSEA

Teas for the queasy

- One of the oldest and perhaps the best remedies proven to allay both nausea and motion sickness. Try a w cup of ginger tea. You can buy ginger teabags or, to make stronger tea yourself, peel the skin from a piece of the root, then chop or grate the yellowish part of the root you have a full teaspoon. Put the gratings in a mug, add a cup of boiling water, cover with a saucer and let it steep for 10 minutes. You can drink the tea when it's still hot or after it has cooled down a bit. Alternatively, try eating a few ginger-nuts or a piece of crystallized ginger.
- Second to ginger is peppermint, which has a calming effect on the lining of the stomach. There are many brands of peppermint tea, sold in teabags or loose-tea form, and you can drink a cup whenever you feel nauseous.

Sip something sweet

- Concentrated sugar is likely to calm a shaky stomach. One recommendation is cola syrup (a concentrate used as a base for homemade fizzy cola drinks), which can be found in some pharmacies. Or try a spoonful of golden syrup or honey.
- Make a homemade anti-nausea syrup. Put half a cup of white sugar with a quarter of a cup of water into a saucepan, turn the heat to medium and stir steadily until you have a clear syrup. After the syrup cools to room temperature, take 2 tablespoons as needed.
- Open a bottle of cola and stir it until it goes flat. Drink it room temperature. Some people swear by flat 7-Up or guns ale, also at room temperature.

CHAPTER TWENTY-NINE

NECK AND SHOULDER PAIN

Heal with heat

- Heat helps to relieve pain, relaxes the muscles reduces joint stiffness and speeds up healing. You can use a heating pad stiffness and speeds up healing. You can on low, a hot-water bottle, an infra-red lamp pack. Or simply take a hot bath or shower.
- Moist heat eases a stiff, sore neck caused by m tension. Make a neck compress by soaking a towel in hot (ma boiling) water. Fold the towel and wring it out well. Unfold and place it over the back of your neck and shoulders the wet towel with a dry one and leave both in place for 10 minutes.
- For easy, fast relief, simply set a hair dryer on warm and blow the air onto your neck.

Apply some pressure

- Try this simple trick: with your thumb or fingertips, apply steady pressure on the painful spot on your neck to 3 minutes. This should lessen your pain significantly.
- A gentle massage can work wonders on neck and pain. Place the fingers of your left hand on your neck just below your ear, and stroke the muscle downward motion towards your collarbone. Do times and repeat on the other side. Using a massage oil lotion to which you have added a few drops of la geranium oil will enhance the soothing effects.

Rub on a liniment

- Apply a cream known as a counter-irritant. These products irritate nerve endings, diverting the brain's attention from the pain. Over the counter brands include the delightfully named Fiery Jack, Algipan and Ralgex.

CHAPTER THIRTY

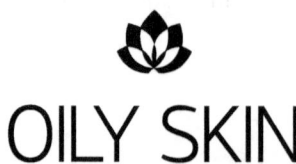

OILY SKIN

Keep your skin clean

- Wash your face with warm water. It dissolves oil more effectively than cool water.
- Choose the right cleanser. Whether you prefer soap bars or liquid cleansers, avoid creamy products such as Dove, that have added moisturizers. Bar soaps like Neutrogena or Simple Soap are perfectly effective, although you can also use cleansers formulated specifically for oily skin (they're likely to be more expensive)
- If you have periodic acne outbreaks, choose a soap formulated for spots, such as Boots ACT wash bar. These discourage the growth of acne-causing bacteria.
- Use a liquid face wash that contains alpha-hydroxy acids (AHAs), such as citric acid, lactic acid or glycolic acid. The AHAs work in several different ways; they help to wash away dead skin cells, they reduce the oil in your pores and they also combat infection.

Make your own toner

- After you've washed your face, soak a cotton pad in witch mazel and dab it all around. Use it twice a day for two to three weeks. After the third week, apply it once a day. Witch hazel contains tannins, which have an astringent effect, making the pores tighten up as they dry.
- Witch hazel contains tannins, which have an astringent effect, making the pores tighten up as they dry.
- The herbs yarrow, sage and peppermint have astringent properties. To make a homemade skin toner that will improve the look and feel of oily skin, put a tablespoon of one of these herbs in a cup, then fill to the top

with boiling water. Leave to steep for 30 minutes. Strain the liquid and let it cool before you dab it on your face. Whatever is left over can be stored. It will say fresh for three days at room temperature, or five days if your keep it in the refrigerator.

CHAPTER THIRTY-ONE

PREGNANCY AILMENTS

Ease fatigue

- Take a half-hour nap each day. When you sleep, make sure that your feet are raised higher than your heart as this helps to take the pressure off your legs. Don't feel guilty about needing to rest: building a baby can be hard work. If you've got a toddler, rest when your child does, and if the child won't nap, put on a Tweenies video, put your feet up and settle down and watch it too.
- Get some exercise every day. Aerobic activity, such as walking or swimming, gives you more energy. And labour and delivery will be easier if you've been exercising regularly.

Deflate swollen feet

- Improve circulation to aching feet with alternating hot and cold footbaths. The hot water brings blood to your feet and the cold moves it back out. Fill two large bowls with water - one comfortably hot, the other cold. Immerse your feet in the hot water for three minutes, then in the cold water for about 30 seconds. Switch backwards and forwards six times, ending with the cold water.
- After your footbaths, rest for at least ten minutes with your feet propped up.

CHAPTER THIRTY-TWO

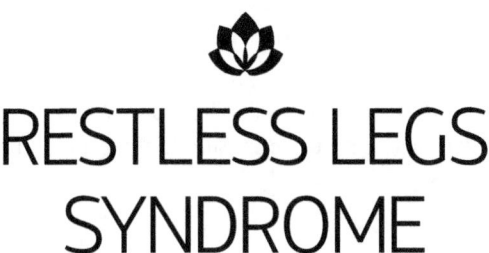

RESTLESS LEGS SYNDROME

Try taking supplements

- Each day, take 800mg calcium and 400mg magnesium, (some naturopaths recommend starting with lower doses, so try 500mg calcium and 250mg magnesium initially - but note that these two minerals must be taken in a 2:1 ratio); plus 800mg potassium. A shortage of any one of these can make legs more twitchy.
- Drink mineral water that's high in magnesium. The optimum magnesium level is in the range of 100mg per litre of water
- Increase your intake of the B vitamin folic acid (also called folate). Folic acid helps to build red blood cells, which in turn help to oxygenate the body. That is an important benefit, as RLS is associated with a decrease in blood oxygen. Food sources of folic acid include leafy green vegetables, orange juice, whole grains and beans. You'll also find folate in most multivitamins.
- Eat iron-rich foods such as dark green vegetables, liver, wheatgerm, kidney beans and lean beef. Iron is part of the myoglobin molecule, which is a protein that stores oxygen in the muscles until it's needed. Without iron, myoglobin can't hold enough oxygen, and muscle problems may develop.

The home stretch

- When you get the urge to move your legs, start rubbing them or stretch them to their full length and point your toes. These intentional movements send signals to your brain that can override the strange

tingling sensations of RLS. But be sure to stop if the stretching causes leg cramps. These suggest a magnesium deficiency, which can't be alleviated by stretching.
- Sit on the edge of the bed and firmly massage your calves to give the muscles deeper stimulation.
- If these treatments don't calm your legs, get up and go for a brief walk around the house or the bedroom. Take long steps and bend your legs to stretch the muscles.

CHAPTER THIRTY-THREE

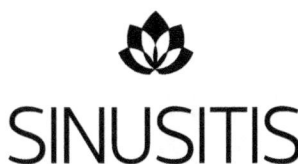

SINUSITIS

Do some steam cleaning

- Steam can relieve painful sinus pressure. Take a long bee shower, inhaling the steam and letting the water spray on your face. Then snort and swallow the hot water until your sinuses are clear.
- Give your congested sinuses a mentholated steam treatment Pour boiling water into a basin and add a few drops of eucalyptus oil. Set the basin on a steady surface (not on your knee or on a bed), then drape a towel over your head and shoulders and lean forwards so that it forms a tent over the basin. Keep your face about 45cm (18in) above the water as you breathe in deeply through your nose. As the vapour rises, it carries tiny droplets of oil into your sinuses and loosens secretions. Do this for as long as is comfortable.
- If you don't have any eucalyptus oil, add a teaspoon of Vicks VapoRub or squeeze a Karvol capsule into the water instead. Sniff a salt solution
- Another method of loosening mucus and reducing swelling is irrigating the sinuses with a saline solution. You can buy the solution from a pharmacy, or make your own by mixing y teaspoon of table salt and a pinch of bicarbonate of soda in a cup of warm water. Then fill a medicine syringe (sold for administering medicines to babies) with the solution. Closing one nostril with your thumb, tilt your head back and squirt the solution into one nostril while you sniff. Blow your nose gently, then repeat with the other nostril.
- You can also use a device called a neti pot, available online and at some health-food shops. (The neti pot is used in Ayurvedic medicine and looks like a small watering can with a narrow spout.) Pour the lukewarm saline solution into one nostril. The liquid will come out of the other nostril. Once it has drained out, blow your nose gently into a tissue. Repeat with

the other nostril using the rest of the saline solution.

CHAPTER THIRTY-FOUR

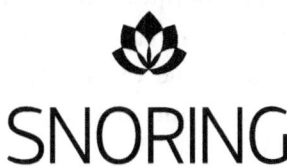

SNORING

Put yourself in a good position

- Buy yourself a few extra pillows and prop yourself up in bed, rather than lying flat on your back. You'll prevent the tissues in your throat from falling into your air passages.
- Raise the head of your bed. An easy way to do it is to place several flat boards under the legs at the top end of the bed. A couple of old phone books under each leg should also raise the bed enough to do the trick.
- Sleep on your side. Of course, there's no guarantee you'll stay in that position, but at least start on your side with your arms wrapped around a pillow. There's a good reason you don't want to sleep on your back: in that position, your tongue and soft palate rest against the back of your throat, blocking the airway.
- If hugging a pillow doesn't help, you can tackle the problem with using a tennis ball. Sew a little pouch onto the back of your pyjama top and tuck a tennis ball inside. At night, if you start to roll onto your back while you're asleep, you'll get a nudge from the ball, prompting you to get back on your side.

Unblock your nose

- If nasal congestion is causing your snoring, try taking a decongestant or antihistamine before you go to bed. But use these only as a temporary measure if you suspect that a cold or allergy is to blame. Prolonged use of either can be harmful.
- Tape your nose open with nasal strips, available at most pharmacies. They may look odd, but who's looking? Following the directions on the package, tape one of the strips to the outside of your nose before you

fall asleep. They work by lifting and opening your nostrils to increase airflow.
- Gargle with a peppermint mouthwash to shrink the lining of your nose and throat. This is especially effective if your snoring is a temporary condition caused by a head cold or an allergy. To mix up the herbal gargle, add 1 drop of peppermint oil to a glass of cold water. (But only gargle - do not swallow.)

CHAPTER THIRTY-FIVE

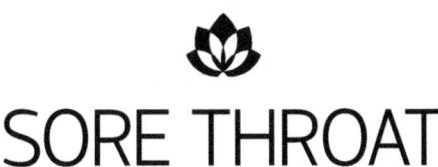

SORE THROAT

Get gargling

- For fast and effective relief, there's nothing to beat an old-fashioned saltwater gargle. Salt acts as a mild antiseptic and also draws water out of mucous membranes in the throat, which helps to clear phlegm. Dissolve / teaspoon of salt in a glass of warm water (use the warmest you can easily tolerate), gargle and spit out. Repeat every hour if it helps.
- For a spicier gargle, add 10-20 drops of Tabasco sauce to a glass of water. Tabasco is made from peppers so it works like capsaicin and it also has anti-viral properties. Don't swallow the gargle as it may irritate the stomach.
- Alternatively, gargle with a bicarbonate of soda solution, using 4 teaspoon of bicarbonate in a glass of warm water. It will soothe inflammation.

The healing power of honey

- Honey has long been used as a sore throat remedy. It has antibacterial properties, which can help to speed up healing. It also acts as a hypertonic osmotic, which means that it draws water out of inflamed tissue. This reduces the swelling and discomfort. Add 2 or 3 teaspoons to a cup of hot water or herbal tea.
- Hot lemon with honey can also relieve pain. Combine the juice of half a lemon with hot water and add two teaspoons of honey. You can add a tablespoon or two of brandy, whisky or ort to this for an appetizing and mildly numbing hot toddy.
- Blackurrant makes another popular and soothing hot drink. The easiest way to make a blackcurrant gargle is to dilute a concentrate such as

Ribena with hot water and sip slowly.

CHAPTER THIRTY-SIX

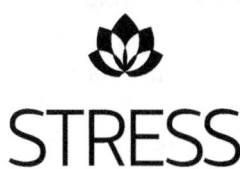

STRESS

Anti-anxiety herbs and supplements

- Ever since ancient Greeks began enjoying camomile tea, it has been praised for its healing properties. Today, when an estimated one million cups are drunk each day throughout the world, herbalists and naturopathic doctors recommend camomile as a wonderful remedy for stress. Drink 1 cup three times a day.
- You can also add camomile, along with other calming herbs such as lavender and valerian, to bathwater for a nervesoothing soak. Wrap the dried herbs in a piece of cheesecloth and hold it under the tap while you fill the bath.
- Get more vitamin C. In one study, people under pressure who took 1000mg of vitamin C a day had milder increases in blood pressure and brought their stress hormone levels back to normal more quickly than people who didn't take it.
- Look to Panax ginseng, a herb valued for its ability to protect the body from stress. It has been shown to balance the release of stress hormones and support the organs that produce them (the pituitary gland, the hypothalamus, and the adrenal glands). Take 100 to 250mg twice a day during times of stress, starting at the lower end of the dosage range and increasing your intake gradually. Experts recommend that you stop taking it for a week every two or three weeks.

Focus your mind

- Relaxing through meditation has been clinically proven to short-circuit stress. Sit in a comfortable position somewhere where you won't be disturbed. Close your eyes. Now choose a word or phrase to focus on

- it's okay', for example. As you concentrate on breathing in and out, repeat the phrase each time you exhale. If you get distracted by other thoughts, gently put them out of your mind and return to your word or phrase. Continue for 10 to 20 minutes. Practise at least once a day.
- Research has found that certain types of music can reduce heart rate, blood pressure and even levels of stress hormones in the blood. Take a break and listen to music you find soothing.
- Do a time-travel exercise. When you're feeling knotted up with some current anxiety, remember something that you felt just as tense about a year ago. How important does it seem today? Now try to project a year into the future and look back on your present dilemma. The chances are, that your 'leap forward' in time will give you a better perspective on what you're going through now.

CHAPTER THIRTY-SEVEN

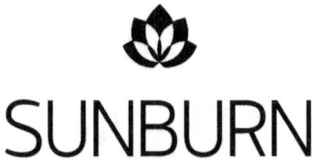

SUNBURN

First, cool it down

- The most important treatment for sunburn is to cool it down, so take cooling measures before you try anything else. Soak any sunburned areas in cold water or with cold compresses for 15 minutes. The cold reduces swelling and wicks away heat from your skin.
- If you're burned all over, take a soak in a cool bath to which you've added oatmeal. You can either buy a colloidal oatmeal product such as Aveeno - which remains in suspension in the bathwater - or finely grind a cup of oats in a food processor and add it to your bath.
- Brew a pot of green tea and let it cool. Soak a cloth in the tea and use it as a compress. Green tea contains ingredients that help to protect the skin from ultraviolet radiation damage and reduce inflammation.
- Use the cooling, aromatic qualities of peppermint to soothe the scorch of sunburn. Either make peppermint tea or mix 2 drops of peppermint oil with a cup of lukewarm water. Chill the concoction and gently bathe the sunburned area using a soft cloth.

CHAPTER THIRTY-EIGHT

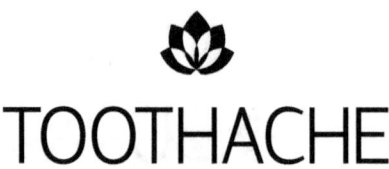

TOOTHACHE

Kill the pain with spices

- Dab some clove oil directly on your bad tooth. Clove oil has remarkable bacteria-slaying properties - and it also has a numbing effect, which is why it's long been used as a remedy for toothache. In the 1800s, when toothpaste was scant and dentists employed tools of torture, every doctor carried a good supply of clove oil. Today it is known that this extract from the clove bud contains eugenol, which acts as a local anaesthetic. The oil may sting at first, but then blissful relief sets in.
- You can get the same numbing effect from whole cloves. Put a few in your mouth, let them moisten until they soften, bruise them a bit between your non-hurting molars to release their oil, then hold the softened cloves against your painful tooth for up to half-an-hour.
- If you don't have any cloves, make a paste with powdered ginger and cayenne pepper. Pour the powdered ingredients in the bottom of a cup, then add a drop or two of water to form the paste. Roll a small ball of cotton into enough paste to saturate it, and place it on your painful tooth. (This mixture can irritate the gums, so you should be careful to keep the cotton only on the tooth.) In addition to using the spices together, you can also try them separately. Either one can help to relieve tooth pain.

Pain relieving mouthwashes

- Rinse your mouth out with a tincture of myrrh. The astringent effects can help with inflammation and myrrh offers the added benefit of killing bacteria. Simmer 1 teaspoon of powdered myrrh in 200ml water for 30 minutes. Strain and let cool. Rinse with a teaspoon of the solution in k cup of water five to six times a day.

- Peppermint tea has a nice flavour and some numbing power. Put a teaspoon of dried peppermint leaves in a cup of boiling water and steep for 20 minutes. After the tea cools, strain it, swish it around in your mouth, then spit it out or swallow. Repeat as often as needed.
- To help to kill bacteria and relieve some discomfort, rinse out with a mouthful of 20 vols hydrogen peroxide solution Hiluted in equal parts with water. This can provide temporary felief if the toothache is accompanied by fever and a horrible faste in the mouth (both are signs of infection), but like other foothache remedies, it is only a stopgap measure until you see your dentist and can get the source of infection investigated And treated. Hydrogen peroxide solution should never be swallowed. Spit it out, then rinse out your mouth several times with ordinary water.
- Stir a teaspoon of salt into a glass of warm water and rinse for up to 30 seconds before you spit it out. Salt water cleanses the area around the tooth and draws out some of the fluid that causes swelling. Repeat this treatment as often as needed.

CHAPTER THIRTY-NINE

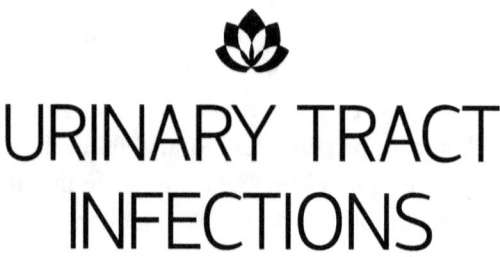

URINARY TRACT INFECTIONS

Drink up

- At the first sign of infection, mix a cold, frothy drink with bicarbonate of soda. Dissolve 1/4 teaspoon of bicarb in 125ml (4fl oz) water. Drink 2 glasses of plain water, then the mixed drink. The bicarb makes the urine less acidic, which reduces the stinging or burning sensation when you pee.
- Throughout the day, drink a glass of water every hour or so. When you flood your urinary tract with water, you flush out bacteria. Also, the more water you drink, the more you dilute your urine, so it's less irritating.
- It's not an old wives' tale: scientific research has shown that cranberry juice really does help women to get rid of urinary tract infections faster. It also helps to prevent them occurring in the first place. There's nothing in the juice to stop bacteria from multiplying, but it contains a chemical that prevents bacteria from sticking to the lining of the urinary tract. And, if bacteria don't stick, they are easily flushed away by your urine. Drink a 300ml (2 pint) glass every day, both as a way to prevent UTIs and to treat them.
- Avoid citrus drinks, tomato juice, coffee and alcohol. All of these drinks may make urination more painful.
- Try these infection-busting teas
- Make a cup of garlic tea. It sounds pretty disgusting, but if you're suffering cystitis pain, you'll try anything. Garlic contains powerful bacteria-killing compounds that make 1 ideal for battling the bugs that cause UTIs. Peel a couple of fresh garlic cloves, mash them well, then

drop them in warn water. Let them steep for five minutes.
- To help your immune system fight the infection - and boost your fluid intake at the same time - make echinacea tea using tea bags or by steeping 2 teaspoons of the raw root in hot water. Drink 3 cups of tea a day.
- Make a tea of lovage (a member of the carrot family) by pouring a cup of boiling water over 2 teaspoons of the minced, dried root. Steep for 10 minutes, then strain and drink. This garden herb contains components with anti-inflammatory and bacteria-killing powers. It's also a diuretic, which helps to flush out the system.
- Try drinking nettle tea. Nettle is a diuretic. It will make you urinate more, which will help to flush bacteria out of your system. Use a teaspoon of the dried herb to a cup of hot water. Drink 1 cup a day.

CHAPTER FORTY

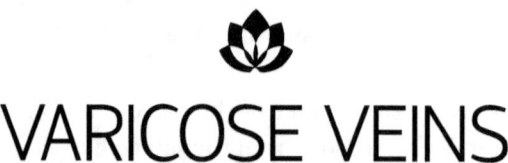

VARICOSE VEINS

Put your feet up

- Lie back on a sofa or armchair, with your legs higher than your heart. Varicosity is the result of blood pooling in your veins, and if you prop up your feet, it lets those 'pools' drain downhill towards your heart. If you're doing the chores at home, take a break from time to time for this couch-potato assignment. Even at work, you may be able to tip back your chair and put your feet up for a while.
- For a more active approach, try this simple yoga move: lie on your back near a wall, propping your feet against the wall with your knees straight so that your legs are at a 45° angle. Hold the position for 3 minutes, breathing deeply and evenly.

Give your veins some help

- For three months, take 250mg of horse chestnut twice a day. A traditional herbal remedy for varicose veins - and one that is recommended by experts today - horse chestnut improves blood vessel elasticity and also seems to strengthen the valves inside veins. After your third month on horse chestnut, take it just once day.
- Take 200mg gotu kola extract three times a day. This herb enhances the strength of blood vessel walls and the connective tissue that surrounds veins. In an Italian study, people who were taking gotu kola showed measurable improvements in the functioning of their veins. Do not take in pregnancy.
- Add some lemon peel to citrus drinks or to your tea. The peel contains a substance called rutin, a type of flavonoid that helps to prevent leakage from small blood vessels.

CHAPTER FORTY-ONE

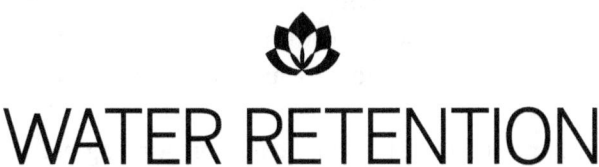

WATER RETENTION

Fight water with water

- It may sound strange but drinking more water could solve the problem of fluid retention. If you're dehydrated, your body stores water to cope with what it sees as a dry spell. Also, when you drink more water, you'll urinate more and pass more salt from your body. Put 2 litres of water in the fridge every morning and try to finish it by the end of the day.

Adjust your salt-potassium balance

- Eat less salt. Most of the salt we eat comes from processed foods, such as soups, sauces, packaged snacks and even shopbought bread. Choose, instead, unprocessed fresh foods such as fruits, vegetables and whole grains that don't come in a box, bag or tin. Make your own bread if you can (a breadmaker is a worthwhile investment). When you do eat processed foods, try to get versions that are labelled 'low salt' or 'low sodium'.
- Get more potassium. This mineral does not work directly as a diuretic, but the right balance of potassium and sodium is crucial for regulating your body's fluid levels. Most people get too little potassium and too much sodium. Eat plenty of fruits and vegetables that are high in potassium, such as bananas, avocados, potatoes, oranges and orange juice. Potassium is also present in high levels in meat, poultry, milk and yoghurt

Flush fluid out the natural way

- Drink 2 to 4 cups of dandelion tea a day. Dandelion leaf is a natural diuretic, allowing your kidneys to drain away more water. The herb is also a rich source of potassium. To make the tea, add 1% tablespoons dried dandelion (available in health food shops) to a litre of water and bring to the boil. Simmer for 15 minutes, strain and let cool before drinking.
- Try drinking nettle tea made from common stinging nettles. Nettle is a natural diuretic. To make the tea, place a heaped teaspoon of powdered root in a cup of cold water. Bring to a boil, boil for 1 minute, then remove from the heat and let steep for 10 minutes. Drink 1 cup four times a day.
- Corn silk is mildly diuretic, possibly because of its high potassium content. Put a teaspoon of dried corn silk (available from some health-food shops and online) in cold water. Boil for 2 to 3 minutes, then strain. Drink 1 cup several times a day. • While you're piling up your plate with fruit and vegetables for their potassium content, save some room for celery, watermelon, asparagus and cucumbers. All contain chemicals that work as natural diuretics.
- The spice turmeric, an ingredient in curry powder, has anti-inflammatory qualities, and may inhibit water retention, according to research in China. Use it freely in your cooking.

CHAPTER FORTY-TWO

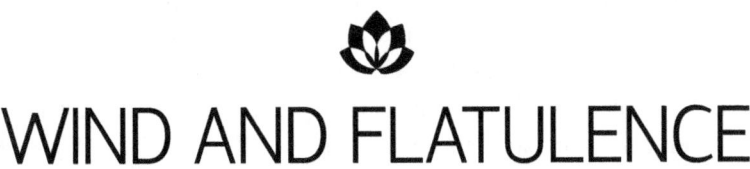

WIND AND FLATULENCE

Deflate your diet

- Certain foods are notorious for producing gas. Avoid them if they give you trouble. They include beans, cabbage, bran, cauliflower, broccoli, onions, prunes, raisins and Brussels sprouts. You could also add eggs to the list, as the sulphur in the yolk contributes to smelly gas.
- Before you cook beans or pulses, soak them overnight. The next day, pour off the old water, then replenish with fresh water for boiling. Even better than boiling for removing gas is to cook beans in a pressure cooker.
- Avoid sugar-free sweets and chewing gums that contain the sweeteners sorbitol, xylitol and mannitol. Your body has trouble digesting them and, when they reach the colon, the resident bacteria there feed on them and produce gas.
- Cut down on fructose, a sugar found in honey, fruit and fruit juices. Like other sweeteners that are difficult to digest, fructose stays in the colon, where bacteria feed on it and create gas. Don't cut whole fruit from your diet but reduce your intake of fruit juice and honey.
- If you're adding more fibre to your diet, do it gradually. Fibre is terrific for your health, but adding a lot to your diet all at once can increase wind.

Look at dairy produce

- Could you be lactose intolerant? Try giving up dairy foods for a few days and see if it makes a difference.

If you are lactose intolerant, you have a low intestinal level of lactase, the enzyme needed to digest lactase, which is a type of sugar found in dairy foods. If you can't bear the thought of giving up milk, you can buy lactase enzyme from pharmacies and add it to milk. Many people who are lactose intolerant can eat hard cheeses such as Swiss cheeses and mature Cheddar. They can usually tolerate yoghurt and buttermilk, as well. Ifcan usually tolerate yoghurt and buttermilk, as well. If you're lactose intolerant, you should also look out for products labelled 'low-lactose' or try soya substitutes

CHAPTER FORTY-THREE

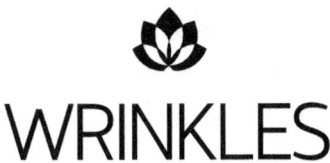

WRINKLES

Smooth fine lines with natural acids

- Use a lotion or cream that contains alpha-hydroxy acids, or AHAs. AHAs come from milk, fruit and sugar cane, and act by clearing away dead cells on the surface of your skin. These products encourage collagen growth, which fills in wrinkles. They also counteract free radicals - rogue oxygen molecules in your body that can damage your skin. Since AHAs can sometimes cause irritation, try rubbing a little of the product on a small patch of skin first. If the patch doesn't turn red by the next day, the moisturizer is safe for you to use.
- Soak a clean flannel in milk and apply it to your skin. Milk contains alpha-hydroxy acids.
- Apply fresh aloe vera gel, which contains malic acid. Cut off a leaf at the base and slit it open. Scrape out the gel with a spoon, taking care not to rupture the green rind, and apply.
- Papayas are full of enzymes that can etch away the top layer of your skin, lessening the appearance of wrinkles. Wash and peel a papaya, then thoroughly mix 2 tablespoons of the pulp with 1 tablespoon of dry oatmeal to help exfoliate your skin. Apply it to your skin and leave it on for 10 minutes. Scrub off the mixture with a flannel.

Soften and moisturize

- Apply a moisturizer every morning after washing to help retain moisture and make your skin feel softer. Look for the moisturizers that also contain sunscreens to protect your skin from ultra-violet rays. Don't forget to apply moisturizer to your neck and hands as well as your face.

- Try an avocado facial. This supplies moisture plus vitamin E, an antioxidant. Puree the pulp, smooth it on your face, and leave it on for 20 minutes.
- Eat, sleep and move for smoother skin
- Eat fish such as salmon, sardines, fresh tuna and mackerel several times a week. These are rich in omega-3 fatty acids, which are very nourishing to your skin.
- Another good way to get omega-3s is to eat a teaspoon of flax seed oil a day. Mix it with juice or pour it over a salad.
- Pile your plate with plenty of fruits, vegetables, nuts and seeds. These provide vitamins A, C, and E - antioxidants that block harmful free radicals before they can cause skin damage.
- As well as getting more vitamin C in your diet, you could go a step further by putting it onto your skin. Recent French research found vitamin C skin cream to be as effective as the current 'gold standard' vitamin A-based retinol creams. Both vitamins A and C are ingredients in several skin creams; if you want to give vitamin C a whirl, look for Reti-C corrective day cream and Reti-C night concentrate.
- Get in the habit of sleeping on your back. When you sleep on your side or stomach, you bury your face in the pillow, 'ironing in' wrinkles and crevices.
- Exercise for 20 to 30 minutes most days of the week. You've probably noticed that exercise can make your skin flush - a sure sign that oxygen and nourishment in your blood are reaching the capillaries in your skin.

The power of prevention

- Don't smoke.
- Drink enough water to make your urine very pale. This really does help to keep your skin moist. . On sunny days, apply a broad-spectrum sunscreen to your face, neck and other areas of exposed skin before you go outdoors, and head for the shade in midday sun.
- Never use a tanning salon. Half-an-hour on a sunbed does more harm than lying on the beach all day without sunscreen.
- Wear sunglasses to avoid crow's feet - wrinkles that come from screwing up your eyes. Even existing crow's feet can fade after several months of consistently wearing sunglasses.

www.ingramcontent.com/pod-product-compliance
Lightning Source LLC
Chambersburg PA
CBHW070822220526
45466CB00002B/738